LOSING WEIGHT WITHOUT DIETING: DISCOVER WEIGHT LOSS SECRETS TO HELP YOU LOSE WEIGHT WITHOUT DIETING

JEFF ANDERSON

Table of Contents

TABLE OF CONTENTS

BEING OVERWEIGHT IS MORE DEADLY THAN YOU THINK

HEALTH RECONSIDERED

SO YOU'RE TELLING ME I CAN EAT WHATEVER, LOSE WEIGHT AND BE HEALTHY?

SELF-CONTROL AND APPETITE REGULATION

THE SAD TRUTH ABOUT THE SUPPLEMENT INDUSTRY

EXERCISE RECOMMENDATIONS FOR LOSING WEIGHT

WHERE'S THE DIET?

STILL NOT LOSING WEIGHT...WHAT SHOULD I DO?

FINAL NOTES

BEING OVERWEIGHT IS MORE DEADLY THAN YOU THINK

With obesity more prevalent now than ever in today's gluttony-encouraging society, it goes without saying that you're not alone of if you're looking to lose that spare tire around your hips. The typical "American" lifestyle generally includes sitting behind a computer for 10 hours a day and mindlessly grazing on calorie-dense, nutrient-devoid foods. Most people don't get much exercise aside from their mighty voyage from the parking lot to the office.

To make matters worse, the health maladies associated with being highly overweight may be just as life-threatening. One of those maladies is the disease diabetes mellitus. 25.8 million children and adults in the United States (8.3% of the population) have diabetes, and that number is increasing at an exponential rate.[1] Moreover, heart disease is the number one cause of death (in the United States), and being overweight is strongly correlated with cardiac consequences.

Most readers likely already knew how dangerous being overweight is, but yet more and more people are becoming obese as time progresses. So why is it exactly that people continue to overeat when the implications can be life threatening? Well, there are a plethora of issues that contribute to overeating, but appetite regulation gone awry is definitely a major culprit; this topic will be discussed further in Chapter 2.

HEALTH RECONSIDERED

Regrettably, the health and fitness realms are led by models/bodybuilders who unbeknownst to the general public lead very unhealthy lifestyles just to look a certain way. A las, that is a diatribe for another time. The good news is that everything you've ever known about dieting and "clean"/healthy eating is pretty much dogmatic nonsense. Read on to learn why that is...

More often than not, people seem to haphazardly throw the word healthy around when it comes to diet and exercise, but the reality is that what is healthy for one individual may or may not be healthy for another. In the Darwinian/biological sense, something that is healthy will serve simply to increase the fitness/survivability of the organism in question. Therefore, a "healthy" food, for example, is simply nourishment that is conducive to longevity.

Ask yourself, "What makes a certain food outright health-promoting?" The first words that pop into most people's mind are usually along the lines of "organic," "natural," "free-range," dairy-free," "sugar-free," "gluten-free," "hormone-free," "low-fat," "low-carb," "low-calorie," the list goes on. Do you see the assumptions being made here? Why is a food that's low-carb or organic, for example, always a healthy choice? Is a food unhealthy because it's been modified or processed in some capacity? The truth is that pretty much every food you find a grocery store is processed to some degree (yes, even "organic" foods), and that doesn't make the food any less healthy than it would be otherwise.

On the flipside, when people think of foods that are unhealthy they likely think of provisions like pizza, burgers, candy and ice cream (aka "junk" food). Why though? Is it because those foods tend to be high in fat and/or sugar and low in micronutrient content? This may come as a surprise, but the fact of the matter is that very few foods/ingredients are wholly unhealthy; it's the amount that you eat those foods in that determines whether or not they are good for you and your goals. Barring specific food allergies and intolerances, or a baseless fear of certain food additives (like artificial sweeteners), there is little basis to label a particular food as being wholly unhealthy.

So you're telling me I can eat whatever, lose weight and be healthy?

Many readers are likely shocked at the previous paragraph. If you read it and thought to yourself, "Wait...This guy is telling me I can eat whatever I want and still meet my health and fitness goals?!" Well, the short answer is "Yes, absolutely." The idea of no foods being off limits often leads "clean" eaters into a frenzy. How can eating things like pizza and ice cream be conducive to health and longevity? Quite simply because if you're not taking in more calories than you're burning throughout the day , than it doesn't really make much of a difference where your energy is coming from.

Literature has shown that the absolute number one factor in losing or gaining bodyweight is total daily energy (calorie) intake versus total daily energy expenditure. That being said, the composition of your diet (aka the macronutrient proportion from which those calories come from) does still matter, just not to as strong of a degree as calorie intake does. This is to say that a diet composed of 1,200 calories coming from carbohydrates only will have different physiological ramifications than a balanced 1,200-calorie diet containing proteins, fats and carbohydrates (more on why this is later on).

The idea of being able to eat any food you want while losing weight may seem like a dream come true because it's often interpreted as, "This guy is saying I can eat cake and donuts ad libitum and still lose weight!" Further from reality that could not be.

What it really means is that you can eat most any food you wish so long as it meets your energy and macronutrient needs at the end of the day. Very few foods/ingredients are outright unhealthy because they are likely beneficial in some capacity.

Don't misinterpret the preceding to mean that you should go drink a gallon of high-fructose corn syrup and think that's going to be healthy, because surely that's not what has been iterated. There is plenty of research that goes into the potential deleterious effects on of things like artificial ingredients and other food additives, but frankly if you're not consuming those things day-in and day-out in copious amounts there is little reason to be concerned about their effects on your health.

Hopefully you can now see the relativity of what makes a food "healthy." When you look at no foods as being "off limits" it creates a whole new dynamic behind dieting. This is very liberating for most people, and ultimately makes them more prone to long-term success on a weight loss regimen.

WHY "DIETING" MAY ACTUALLY BE RUINING YOUR WEIGHT-LOSS EFFORTS

Much to the chagrin of many individuals, dietary restriction can actually worsen weight management issues. A few studies have looked at how both exposure techniques and training can help improve eating behavior self-control in individuals looking to lose weight. The results suggest that while dietary restraint can be useful to an extent, an eating plan that is pliable/flexible with regards to food selection is more prone to healthy long-term weight management.[2,3]

Diets that present harsh stipulations and/or greatly restrict specific nutrients fail in the long-term due to their impractical demands and lack of balance. This is why many people that try the Atkins Diet (which is a diet that promotes greatly restricting carbohydrate intake) don't last more than a few days before they give in and binge on high-sugar foods. That's how pretty much everyone will react if they go from eating anything they want to being in a position where they're only supposed to eat the same certain, limited selection of foods everyday.

Make no mistake about it, binge eating can and will wreak havoc on your body and psychological connection with food. This is why a diet that doesn't restrict you will be more successful in the long run because you won't feel inhibited all the time. When you think about the biological basis for eating, it really boils down to being something that sustains us, and nourishes us, both mentally and physically. The idea that you have to sacrifice taste and psychological enjoyment of your diet to achieve the body of your dreams is flat out hogwash.

Now, before moving on it is imperative to iterate that self-control is still going to be necessary if you want to lose weight and keep it off. Many people may not have the level of discipline necessary to enjoy certain foods they crave in moderation, but the good news is there are ways around that conundrum (which will be covered in the following section).

Self-control and Appetite Regulation

Many readers may feel that they lack the requisite discipline to flourish on a diet (especially when the idea of enjoying foods they genuinely enjoy is considered). While most of your ability to control yourself when indulging on foods you like is relegated to your willpower (you are, after all, human), some of it is also influenced by your appetite.

There seems to be a lack of understanding behind the terms *appetite* and *hunger.* Appetite is used to describe the psychological desire to eat food, whereas hunger is the body signaling the physiological need for food. While both appetite and hunger have their own designations, there is certainly interplay between them and one can influence the other.

So for example, if you eat a well-sized meal then you should no longer be hungry. However, if all the sudden you get a sweet tooth for ice cream, that is your appetite (psychological desire) kicking in.

The reason your appetite may be high despite your hunger being satisfied is likely due to a disconnection between your brain and your stomach. Various hormones secreted in the human body act as neuromodulators that influence cognitive behavior towards appetite (or lack thereof).

The primary hormone responsible for stimulating hunger is called ghrelin, secreted in the pancreas and stomach. Shortly after you start eating food, various hormones such as leptin and cholecystokinin start to secrete satiety/fullness signals that communicate with the brain and tell you you're getting full.

This is why it is advised to eat your food slowly so your brain has time to catch up with your stomach, so to speak. Here are some more appetite regulation suggestions that should help decrease your desire for that late-night pint of chocolate ice cream.

Eat slower—this is a pretty rudimentary tip because it's based on basic physiology; as mentioned earlier in this chapter, eating slowly gives your brain and gut time to connect and recognize you're filling up

Eat foods that provide more satiety early in your meals/day:

- *Fibrous vegetables/fruits* are micronutrient-dense, lower-calorie options that provide bulk to waste in the intestines, hence you feel fuller.

- *Hi-water content foods* such as soups, low-fat dairy, beans, lean meats, poultry, fish, fruits, veggies and certain cooked grains are generally lower in calorie density. Essentially, you get more "bang for your buck" with these options because the water promotes fullness and adds volume to your food.

When in doubt, opt for lower-carb foods and more protein and fats--fats and protein are much more satiating per gram than most carbohydrate sources, so it is to your benefit to emphasize them. Moreover, by lowering carb intake a bit you will reduce blood-sugar swings and keep insulin levels down, both positive things when you are trying to lose bodyweight.

Drink ample amounts of water (or other low-calorie liquids)—the benefits of staying hydrated are rather numerous, and keeping enough liquid in your stomach while you eat can create a sense of fullness (not to mention it's good for digestive purposes).

Get your mind off of food—seems pretty intuitive, but when you sense a hunger pang coming on the last thing you want to do is be around the kitchen when mama is whipping up her famous banana cream pie. Try and keep yourself preoccupied with other things and you'll notice you stop worrying about food so much.

Moderation is key--avoid extremes if possible; don't fall into the trap of restricting yourself to certain foods; enjoy your life a little bit! If you want some pizza, have a slice or two. If you want a slice of cake it won't kill you, just don't eat the whole cake...

Eat until you are just about full and then stop--The fact of the matter is that when you're trying to lose fat, you will undoubtedly be a bit hungry at times. This is normal, your body is being underfed so it will send the signal that it wants more food. Over time though this will subside.

Manage stress/anxiety—many people are likely aware of "stress eating" which seems to be a common occurrence in depressed individuals. On the same token, some people may deal with stress and anxiety by avoiding food. It can only be of benefit for you to manage your stress/anxiety so before eating try and have a calm, pleasant mood which will usually positively affect your appetite regulation.

Get adequate sleep—even acute losses of sleep have been shown to have a host of deleterious effects in humans, including tendency to overeat the next day and concomitant decreases in insulin sensitivity, two things that spell disaster when combined.[11] Sleep loss usually results in feeling stressed out as well, which as aforementioned is generally not favorable for good appetite regulation.

Plan/prep your meals ahead of time--planning your meals ahead of time and knowing what you're going to eat will usually reduce the urge to snack on foods or drink liquids that are high in calories.

SUPPLEMENTAL APPETITE SUPPRESSANTS

Chromium—A trace biological mineral that is purported to improve carbohydrate metabolism and increase serotonin levels as well as decrease serum cortisol levels, which are all positives when seeking appetite suppression.[4] The polynicotinate form is preferred as it is more bioavailable.

5-Hydroxytryptophan (5-HTP) — intermediate metabolite between L-tryptophan and serotonin. Generally extracted from the plant *Griffonia simplicifoli*. The theory here is that serotonin eases stress and thus appetite will be reduced since many people "stress eat".[5]

Caffeine/Synephrine/Yohimbine—these are all stimulant based compounds that should only be used in moderation; for appetite-suppressing purposes it is generally advised to use non-stimulants around meal times and save these for times around your workout.

Glucomannan--a soluble and highly viscous dietary fiber derived from the root of the elephant yam or konjac plant. Studies have shown significant benefits in promoting satiety and improved lipid profiles.[6]

Hoodia—a bit more underwhelming than the other compounds listed here as the studies have haven't really proven hoodia's efficacy in nominal doses.[7] If you can find it cheap then it may be worth a try.

White Kidney Bean Extract—a relatively new compound in the supplement world that is purported to have anorexigenic activity via inhibition of alpha-amylase.[8]

The doses necessary for appetite suppression will vary for many individuals so please follow the label instructions when starting any of these supplements.

THE SAD TRUTH ABOUT THE SUPPLEMENT INDUSTRY

The previous supplemental recommendations are meant more as an alternative plan to the "natural" ways you can suppress your appetite. The supplement industry is unfortunately not one of high integrity. Most companies that produce supplements are simply in it for the money. Unfortunately, this comes at the expense of the consumer's health and hard-earned money. Not only do many supplement companies blatantly lie on their labels about what is in their product, they often include ingredients that have little-to-no scientific validity about their efficacy. Think about it this way, would you trust your doctor if he prescribed you a drug that hasn't even been put through FDA trials or been confirmed to treat the condition it claims to?

You should never be ingesting a product that contains bunk ingredients; it's analogous to flushing money down the toilet (except this is worse for your health). Don't fall prey to quackery, like products that claim to help you lose 20lbs in 4 weeks. There is nothing healthy that will do that for you. Most all supplements that are efficacious and scientifically-proven will need to be used consistently to notice much of the desired benefits. Hype is not real; science is.

Much to the chagrin of many supplement consumers, companies often sacrifice quality just to make products sound elaborate and flashy. For example, a common scheme you may notice is when a company "label dresses" a product by using inferior forms of common ingredients (like zinc oxide in zinc supplements) and/or load it up with negligible amounts of other compounds. To the untrained eye, this makes the product seem worthwhile and high-quality because they can list numerous ingredients on their label. The reality is that they are simply cutting their costs and giving the consumer a useless supplement.

Moreover, few companies seem to actually test their products for impurities and contamination, nor do they source their raw materials from legitimate manufacturers. It's quite vexing to think that so many products are out there that look so nice and flashy on the outside, but what's inside is likely loaded with fillers, dyes, and possible contaminants like mercury.

Just be careful with what supplements you buy and remember that more money doesn't necessarily mean you're getting a superior-quality product.

EXERCISE RECOMMENDATIONS FOR LOSING WEIGHT

Hopefully this chapter doesn't come as a surprise to you...you didn't really think that you were going to be able to lose weight by eating anything and sitting on the couch all day did you? If it was that easy, then you wouldn't be reading this!

Now the good news is that you don't have to beat yourself to death with grueling 3-hour workouts just to lose weight. All you really have to do is a few diligent resistance training sessions per week along with a few bouts of cardiovascular exercise. There is strong evidence that a fitness regimen consisting of a minimum of 3 hours of moderate-intensity (or 2 hours of vigorous-intensity) exercise, with no more than two consecutive non-training days per week, can have significant benefits on insulin sensitivity and improve body composition.

Moreover, cardiovascular exercise, especially high-intensity interval training (HIIT) appears to provide many of the same benefits associated with resistance training. Thus, it's wise for overweight individuals to incorporate both resistance training and cardiovascular exercise (preferably HIIT) in their fitness regimen. An example weekly fitness regimen for someone looking to lose weight might look like this:

Mon/Wed/Fri—45 minutes moderate-intensity weight training

Tue/Thu/Sat—cardiovascular exercise; no need to be excessive with this however it should be 40-50 minutes for low-intensity, steady-state cardio (like a brisk walk) or 15-20 minutes for HIIT (see below for an example of this type of workout):

- Find a hill that is about 50-60 yards long

- Sprint as hard as you can to the top of the hill (should take about 10-15 seconds)

- Walk slowly back down to the bottom of the hill for "active recovery"

- Catch your breath and repeat ten times

Obviously the specific routine/exercises you choose to do should be adjusted to fit your specific goals. Ultimately, the main thing is to just make sure you're doing some form of diligent exercise and being consistent. It cannot be emphasized enough the importance of being consistent about your fitness regimen; keep moving and you're almost certainly going to notice improvements in body composition and feel better about yourself.

Where's the diet?

So if you've made it to this point you may wondering, "Where is the diet plan? Do I just eat whatever I want?" The short answer to that is, "Yes." However, a few assumptions are being made here. It is assumed that you're reading this book since you're looking to lose weight without changing your eating habits. It is also assumed that you DO NOT currently exercise. Read on and this will be addressed...

Logically speaking, your body will only lose weight if you are burning more calories than you eat on a daily basis. This is something that you cannot work you way around. The reason that you won't be needing to change your dietary habits (much) is because you will be exercising (using the recommendations in Chapter 3) and burning several hundred additional calories per day that you haven't been burning in the past.

Now, the main issue is if you have already been exercising diligently and still not lost weight (or worse yet, you're gaining weight without intending too) then the prudent thing to do is simply start skipping breakfast. Many people may think that sounds detrimental but intermittent fasting (i.e. not eating for 12-14 hours) actually works wonders when people can't get over a weight-loss plateau.

Just because you skip breakfast doesn't mean you will feel less energetic or less alert either. In fact, most people who switch from eating breakfast everyday to skipping it and waiting until lunch time to eat their first meal of the day will notice that they actually have more energy and a heightened sense of wellbeing throughout the day.

STILL NOT LOSING WEIGHT...WHAT SHOULD I DO?

If you have been consistently exercising and notice that your weight hasn't dropped much after the first week or two (and you've also implemented the breakfast-skipping tactic) then there are two options: either start tracking your food intake for up to one week and actually see how many calories you eat per day OR skip both breakfast and lunch each day and see how your body reacts.

Skipping breakfast and lunch may seem like a daunting task for many, but remember you will be able to eat bigger portions later in the day. Some people like that idea as it lets them go about their day without worrying about food and then they can go home and have a nice big dinner and a snack later at night and still lose weight. It's a very simple way to reduce calorie intake.

Now if you choose the first option of tracking your food intake, it is recommended to use an online basal metabolic rate (BMR) calculator and compare your calorie intake versus your calorie expenditure. It is very likely that despite exercising consistently you're still eating too much and may have to cut back on portion sizes just a bit. Don't worry, just reduce the serving sizes a tad from each meal and ease your way into it. Also be sure to use the appetite suppression tactics in Chapter 2 to help you control your cravings, should they arise.

A last thing to note is that you can add more cardiovascular exercise into your regimen if you want to, but do not overdo it. It is not good in the long run to overwork yourself with excessive amounts of cardiovascular exercise as this will actually lower your BMR and make you more prone to weight regain. Remember, the goal isn't just to lose weight; it's to lose weight and keep it off!

FINAL NOTES

Thank you for downloading my book, Losing Weight without Dieting: Discover Weight Loss Secrets to Help You Lose Weight without Dieting! I hope you put everything you have learned to use and obtain the body you have always wanted.

If you enjoyed my book and wish to help me out, you can leave the book an honest review on Amazon.

You can check out some of my other health and fitness books by visiting my author page.

Here are some of the other books I have written:

Lose Weight Fast: 101 Ways to Lose up to 10 Pounds in 7 Days

Weight Loss for Women Over 50: The Ultimate Weight Loss Guide to Look and Feel Young Again

References

1. Diabetes Statistics - American Diabetes Association. (n.d.). American Diabetes Association Home Page - American Diabetes Association. http://www.diabetes.org/diabetes-basics/diabetes-statistics/?loc=DropDownDB-stats

2. Johnson, F., Pratt, M., & Wardle, J. (2012). Dietary restraint and self-regulation in eating behavior. *International Journal of Obesity*, *36*(5), 665-674.

3. Smith, C. F., Williamson, D. A., Bray, G. A., & Ryan, D. H. (1999). Flexible vs. Rigid dieting strategies: relationship with adverse behavioral outcomes.*Appetite*, *32*(3), 295-305.

4. Komorowski JR, Tuzcu M, Sahin N, Juturu V, Orhan C, Ulas M, Sahin K. Chromium picolinate modulates serotonergic properties and carbohydrate metabolism in a rat model of diabetes. Biol Trace Elem Res. 2012 Oct;149(1):50-6. doi: 10.1007/s12011-012-9393-x. Epub 2012 Mar 22. PubMed PMID: 22434381.

5. Halford JC, Harrold JA, Lawton CL, Blundell JE. Serotonin (5-HT) drugs: effects on appetite expression and use for the treatment of obesity. Curr Drug Targets. 2005 Mar;6(2):201-13. Review. PubMed PMID: 15777190.

6. Keithley J, Swanson B. Glucomannan and obesity: a critical review. Altern Ther Health Med. 2005 Nov-Dec;11(6):30-4. Review. PubMed PMID: 16320857.

7. Whelan AM, Jurgens TM, Szeto V. Case report. Efficacy of Hoodia for weight loss: is there evidence to support the efficacy claims? J Clin Pharm Ther. 2010 Oct;35(5):609-12. doi: 10.1111/j.1365-2710.2009.01116.x. PubMed PMID: 20831685.

8. Hypoglycaemic and anorexigenic activities of an a-amylase inhibitor from white kidney beans (Phaseolus vulgaris) in Wistar rats, British Journal of Nutrition (2004), 92, 785–790.

9. Hordern, M. D., Dunstan, D. W., Prins, J. B., Baker, M. K., Singh, M. A. F., & Coombes, J. S. (2012). Exercise prescription for patients with type 2 diabetes and pre-diabetes: a position statement from Exercise and Sport Science Australia. *Journal of Science and Medicine in Sport, 15*(1), 25-31.

10. Mendes, R., Sousa, N., Garrido, N., Rocha, P., José, L. T. B., & Victor, M. R. (2013). EFFICACY OF ACUTE HIGH-INTENSITY INTERVAL TRAINING IN LOWERING GLYCEMIA IN PATIENTS WITH TYPE 2 DIABETES: DIABETES EM MOVIMENTO® PILOT STUDY. *British journal of sports medicine*, *47*(10), e3-e3

11. Benedict C, Brooks SJ, O'Daly OG, Almèn MS, Morell A, Åberg K, Gingnell M, Schultes B, Hallschmid M, Broman JE, Larsson EM, Schiöth HB. Acute sleep deprivation enhances the brain's response to hedonic food stimuli: an fMRI study. J Clin Endocrinol Metab. 2012 Mar;97(3):E443-7. doi: 10.1210/jc.2011-2759. Epub 2012 Jan 18. PubMed PMID: 22259064..

www.ingramcontent.com/pod-product-compliance
Lightning Source LLC
Chambersburg PA
CBHW071302280526
45788CB00004B/1813